Log Book for

Pediatric Postgraduates

425/-

AF675108

Log Book for
Pediatric Postgraduates

(As Per NMC Guidelines for Competency-based Postgraduate Training)

Editor

Shetanshu Srivastava

MD MAMS FISMN

Additional Professor

Department of Pediatrics

Dr Ram Manohar Lohia Institute of Medical Sciences

Lucknow, Uttar Pradesh, India

Co-Editor

SN Singh

MBBS MD

Professor and Head

Department of Pediatrics

King George's Medical University

Lucknow, Uttar Pradesh, India

Forewords

Piyush Gupta
Mahima Mittal

JAYPEE

JAYPEE BROTHERS MEDICAL PUBLISHERS

The Health Sciences Publisher

New Delhi | London

JAYPEE **Jaypee Brothers Medical Publishers (P) Ltd**

Headquarters
EMCA House, 23/23-B
Ansari Road, Daryaganj
New Delhi 110 002, India
Landline: +91-11-23272143, +91-11-23272703
+91-11-23282021, +91-11-23245672
e-mail: jaypee@jaypeebrothers.com

Corporate Office
4838/24, Ansari Road, Daryaganj
New Delhi 110 002, India
Phone: +91-11-43574357
Fax: +91-11-43574314
e-mail: jaypee@jaypeebrothers.com

Overseas Office
JP Medical Ltd
83 Victoria Street, London
SW1H 0HW (UK)
Phone: +44-20 3170 8910
e-mail: info@jpmedpub.com

EU GPSR Authorised Representative
Logos Europe, 9 rue Nicolas Poussin
17000, La Rochelle, France
Phone: +33 (0) 6 67 93 73 78
e-mail: contact@logoseurope.eu

Website: www.jaypeebrothers.com
Website: www.jaypeedigital.com

© 2026, Jaypee Brothers Medical Publishers

The views and opinions expressed in this book are solely those of the original contributor(s)/author(s) and do not necessarily represent those of editor(s) or publisher of the book.

All rights reserved. No part of this publication may be reproduced, stored or transmitted in any form or by any means, electronic, mechanical, photocopying, recording or otherwise, without the prior permission in writing of the publishers.

All brand names and product names used in this book are trade names, service marks, trademarks or registered trademarks of their respective owners. The publisher is not associated with any product or vendor mentioned in this book.

Medical knowledge and practice change constantly. This book is designed to provide accurate, authoritative information about the subject matter in question. However, readers are advised to check the most current information available on procedures included and check information from the manufacturer of each product to be administered, to verify the recommended dose, formula, method and duration of administration, adverse effects and contraindications. It is the responsibility of the practitioner to take all appropriate safety precautions. Neither the publisher nor the author(s)/editor(s) assume any liability for any injury and/or damage to persons or property arising from or related to use of material in this book.

This book is sold on the understanding that the publisher is not engaged in providing professional medical services. If such advice or services are required, the services of a competent medical professional should be sought.

Every effort has been made where necessary to contact holders of copyright to obtain permission to reproduce copyright material. If any have been inadvertently overlooked, the publisher will be pleased to make the necessary arrangements at the first opportunity.

Inquiries for bulk sales may be solicited at: jaypee@jaypeebrothers.com

Log Book for Pediatric Postgraduates

First Edition: **2026**

ISBN: 978-93-7202-413-5

Printed in India at Sterling Graphics Pvt. Ltd.

Dedicated to

*The future healers of children—May your knowledge be deep,
your skills be precise, your heart be compassionate,
and your commitment to the well-being of every child remain unwavering*

Contributors

Arvind Kumar Shukla
Assistant Professor
Department of Pediatrics
Maharaja Suhel Dev Autonomous State Government Medical College
Bahraich, Uttar Pradesh, India

Asish Verma
Professor
Department of Pediatrics
Career Institute of Medical Sciences
Lucknow, Uttar Pradesh, India

Dipti Agarwal
Professor
Department of Pediatrics
Dr Ram Manohar Lohia Institute of Medical Sciences
Lucknow, Uttar Pradesh, India

Shetanshu Srivastava
Additional Professor
Department of Pediatrics
Dr Ram Manohar Lohia Institute of Medical Sciences
Lucknow, Uttar Pradesh, India

SN Singh
Professor and Head
Department of Pediatrics
King George's Medical University
Lucknow, Uttar Pradesh, India

Sunil Kumar Rao
Professor
Department of Pediatrics
Banaras Hindu University
Varanasi, Uttar Pradesh, India

Utkarsh Bansal
Professor
Department of Pediatrics
Hind Institute of Medical Sciences
Lucknow, Uttar Pradesh, India

Yashwant Kumar Rao
Professor
Department of Pediatrics
Ganesh Shankar Vidyarthi Memorial Medical College
Kanpur, Uttar Pradesh, India

Foreword

It is a great pleasure to introduce this book for pediatric residents, a comprehensive tool designed to guide, assess, and reflect the professional growth of future pediatricians. In today's rapidly evolving medical field, it is not enough to gain theoretical knowledge; clinical skills, professional behavior, and reflective practices are equally vital components in producing well-rounded, capable healthcare providers.

The book is a testament to the shift toward *"Competency-based Medical Education (CBME)"*, where the focus is on ensuring that learners acquire and demonstrate essential competencies at various stages of their training. Rather than relying solely on traditional methods of assessment, this approach promotes continuous learning, allowing residents to document and reflect upon their experiences. The incorporation of self-assessment and regular faculty feedback further ensures that trainees are actively engaged in their own educational development, fostering a sense of accountability and growth.

The book covers a broad range of competencies, from clinical skills in handling common pediatric conditions to interpersonal communication and professionalism. Residents will also be encouraged to participate in reflective practice, where they critically evaluate their performance and identify areas for improvement. This self-directed learning approach helps to cultivate a lifelong commitment to excellence in patient's care.

I am confident that this book will serve as a valuable tool in enhancing the training of pediatric residents, ensuring that they not only meet the required competencies but also become compassionate, ethical, and skilled pediatricians.

It is my sincere hope that this book will be used not just as a record of skills and experiences but as a roadmap for personal and professional growth, guiding residents toward becoming leaders in the field of pediatrics.

Piyush Gupta
MD FAMS FRCPCH
Former Principal, Professor and Head
Department of Pediatrics
University College of Medical Sciences
New Delhi, India
President, Indian Academy of Pediatrics (2021)

Foreword

It is both an honor and a privilege to introduce the book. Curated by a team of experienced pediatric educators, this essential resource is designed to support the next generation of pediatricians as they embark on their journey through the complex and rewarding field of child health. This book serves not only as a record of learners' clinical experiences but also as a vital tool for reflection, learning, and professional growth during their postgraduate training.

"Training in Pediatrics" is a journey of both personal and professional development. Each entry in this book represents a stepping stone on the path to becoming a competent and compassionate pediatrician. I will encourage learners to use this space to reflect on challenges faced, successes achieved, and lessons learned and to embrace the opportunity to document not just what you did, but how those experiences shaped your approach to patient's care. I also believe that this book encourages collaboration among peers and mentors. Sharing insights and experiences fosters a rich learning environment that enhances clinical practice.

The book is designed as a vital tool to complement the competency-based curriculum for pediatric residents. By integrating a variety of competencies, the book encourages residents to engage deeply with their learning. It emphasizes critical skills such as communication, empathy, and clinical decision-making, which are essential in pediatrics. The book also promotes self-directed learning, pushing residents to identify their educational needs and seek resources accordingly. By adhering to this structured approach, residents will be better prepared to meet the challenges of pediatric practice, ultimately benefiting the children and families they serve. The book not only aligns with current educational standards but also sets a foundation for lifelong learning in the field of pediatrics.

Lastly, dear learners, as you fill these pages with your experiences, insights, and reflections, remember that each entry is a step toward becoming an exceptional pediatrician. Embrace the challenges ahead with enthusiasm and dedication; the future of pediatric care is bright because of your commitment.

Warm regards,

Mahima Mittal MD
Dean (Academics) and Head
Department of Pediatrics
All India Institute of Medical Sciences
Gorakhpur, Uttar Pradesh, India

Preface

Pediatrics requires strong theoretical knowledge along with the skillful, compassionate, and ethical application of that knowledge in varied clinical settings. With the advent of competency-based medical education (CBME) as mandated by the National Medical Commission (NMC), the focus has shifted toward holistic training that integrates clinical expertise, communication skills, professionalism, and reflective practice.

This *Log Book for Pediatric Postgraduates (As Per NMC Guidelines for Competency-based Postgraduate Training)* has been designed as a comprehensive tool to record, monitor, and assess the progressive acquisition of essential competencies during postgraduate training. It serves not only as a repository of clinical encounters, procedures, academic activities, and research milestones, but also as a framework for structured feedback and self-directed learning.

The structured format will help postgraduate residents systematically document their experiences, assess their strengths and limitations, and plan for targeted improvement. It is our hope that this book becomes a companion in the journey of growth, inspiring commitment to lifelong learning and excellence in pediatric care.

Shetanshu Srivastava
SN Singh

Acknowledgments

We extend our sincere gratitude to the National Medical Commission for providing clear guidelines for competency-based postgraduate training, which served as the foundation for this book's design. Our heartfelt thanks go to our esteemed colleagues, faculty members, and postgraduate residents whose valuable suggestions helped refine the structure and content of this book.

We are deeply grateful to Dr Piyush Gupta and Dr Mahima Mittal for their encouraging forewords and for their unwavering dedication to advancing pediatric education in India. We also thank our respective institutions—Dr Ram Manohar Lohia Institute of Medical Sciences, Lucknow, Uttar Pradesh, India, and King George's Medical University, Lucknow—for their support and for fostering an environment of academic excellence.

Lastly, we acknowledge the team at M/s Jaypee Brothers Medical Publishers (P) Ltd, New Delhi, India, for their meticulous efforts in bringing this work to publication. Without the collective dedication of educators, clinicians, and learners, this initiative would not have been possible.

Suggested Reading

1. Aulakh, Roosy & Chhatwal, Jugesh & Dhir, Shashi & Gupta, Priyanka & Gupta, Piyush & Singh, Tejinder. (2021). Postgraduate Logbook. 10.13140/RG.2.2.14722.61120.
2. https://www.iscp.ac.uk/static/public/DOPSJul2015.pdf
3. Mini-CEX form can be downloaded from https://www.abim.org/Media/qlvp1fhb/mini-cex.pdf
4. National Medical Commission. Competency Based Postgraduate Training Programme for MD in Paediatrics. D 11011/1/22/AC/Guidelines/14.05-08-2022. Available from: https://www.nmc.org.in
5. NMC MD Pediatrics Curriculum can be downloaded from https://www.nmc.org.in/wp-content/uploads/2019/09/MD-Pediatrics.pdf
6. Objective Structured Long Examination Record (OSLER) may be used for assessment available at: http://pad.org.pk/forms/OSLER.pdf

Department of Pediatrics

Name :..

Photo

Date of Joining :..

Admission No :..

NMC Registration No :..

Address :..

....

....

Email/Mobile no : ....

Thesis Topic : ....

: ....

Thesis Supervisor : ....

: ....

Department of Pediatrics

Certificate

Certified that the content of this Log Book is the Bonafide work of

Dr.., Postgraduate...

Student of Department of Pediatrics of ....
of...for the academic year...

Signature

Name & Seal of Guide

Signature

Name & Seal of HOD

Index

S. no	Contents
1.	Orientation Program Introduction to Resiliency Training Soft Skills Training Time Management Skills Certifiable Skills
2.	Academic Sessions (a) Case Presentation (b) Seminar (c) Journal Clubs (d) Mortality Meet (e) Quiz
3.	Formative Assessment Workplace Assessment (a) Mini-Clinical Evaluation Exercises (Mini-CEX) (b) Direct Observation of Procedural Skills (DOPS) (c) Case-based Discussion (d) Counseling Skills
4.	Research Skills: Thesis (a) Protocol Presentation (b) Thesis Progress (c) Research Projects (d) Paper/Poster Presentation/Publications
5.	Teaching (a) Undergraduate (b) Staff Training (c) Parents Awareness Programs
6.	Participation in National Days and Weeks Photographs
7.	Self-directed Learning
8.	Professionalism and Ethics
9.	Others Administrative Responsibilities Awards and Honors Testimonials

Orientation Program

Date	Topic/Session	Facilitator	Reflection

Certifiable Skills

Skills	Dates
BLS	
NRP	
PALS	
Basic Course in Biomedical Research	
Biomedical Waste Management	
Course in Ethics Good Clinical Practice	
Safe Injection Practices	
Medicolegal essentials	
Others	
a.	
b.	
c.	
d.	
Proficiency certificate	

Summary of Procedures Done

Observed (0), Perform under supervision (PS), Perform independently (PI)

Year, Month	LP	Surfactant Administration	Exchange Transfusion	Intubation/ Ventilation	TPN	Central Line	Arterial Cannula	Umbilical Cannula	Intraosse-ous cannula	Ascitic Tap	ICD	Peritone-al Dialysis	Biopsy		Bone Marrow Aspirate
													Liver	Kidney	
1st Year															
1															
2															
3															
4															
5															
6															
7															
8															
9															
10															
11															
12															
2nd Year															
1															
2															
3															
4															
5															
6															
7															
8															
9															
10															
11															
12															
3rd Year															
1															
2															
3															
4															
5															
6															
7															
8															
9															
10															
11															
12															

Achieved Skills O-Observe P-PS-Perform under supervision Q-PI-Perform independently	1st Year	2nd Year	3rd Year
1. HEADSS screening (Adolescence)			
2. DDST screening (Development Assessment)			
3. Assessment of Sexual Maturity using Tanner's			
4. M-CHAT-R screening (Autism Assessment)			
5. GMSCF Assessment of Motor Disability (Cerebral Palsy)			
6. Triage: Rapid assessment of ABC			
7. C-ACT (Asthma Assessment)			
8. Hammersmith infant neurological assessment (HINE)			

Postings Details

S. No	Date		Total Duration	Area of Posting	Overall; Performance** (B/M/E)	Unit Incharge Signature
	From	To				

S. No	Date		Total Duration	Area of Posting	Overall; Performance** (B/M/E)	Unit Incharge Signature
	From	To				

	Date					
	From	To				

Including District Postings, Elective Postings and Posting in other Departments, if any.
**Grading: B: Below Expectations, M: Meets Expectations, E: Exceeds Expectations

Participation in Academic Activities

	Attended/Presented												Faculty Signature
	1st Year												
Case-based Discussion													
Seminars													
Journal Club													
Case Presentation													
Tutorial/Symposium													
Workshop/CME													
Inter-Departmental Presentation													
Mortality Meet													
Quiz													
	2nd Year												
Months													
Case-based Discussion													
Seminars													
Journal Club													
Case Presentation													
Tutorial/Symposium													
Workshop/CME													
Inter-Departmental Presentation													
Mortality Meet													
Quiz													
	3rd Year												
Months													
Case-based Discussion													
Seminars													
Journal Club													
Tutorial/Symposium													
Workshop/CME													
Inter-Departmental Presentation													
Mortality Meet													
Quiz													

(a) Case Presentations

S. No	Date	Provisional Diagnosis/Problem	Presented/Attended Write P/A	Moderator's Signature (OSLER Grading P+/P/P-)

*Objective Structured Long Examination Record (OSLER) may be used for assessment available at http://pad.org.pk/forms/OSLER.pdf
^Case-based Analysis and Interpretation; Once a week

Reflections

Date: .... Diagnosis:
What happened?
So what?
What next?
Faculty's Signature Date...

Reflections

Date: ....   Diagnosis:
What happened?
So what?
What next?
Faculty's Signature Date..

Reflections

Date: ....

Diagnosis:

What happened?

So what?

What next?

Faculty's Signature

Date...

Case Presentations

S. No	Date	Provisional Diagnosis/Problem	Presented/Attended Write P/A	Moderator's Signature (OSLER Grading P+/P/P-)

Reflections

Date: ....   Diagnosis:
What happened?
So what?
What next?
Faculty's Signature Date...

(b) Seminars

S. No	Date	Topic	Presented/Attended Write P/A	Moderator's Signature

Seminar Assessment

Date:.................. **Topic:....................................**

Please rate each criterion. All scores of BE must be justified in the comments box. Write U/C if Unable to Comment/Not Observed.

S. No	Criteria	Below Expectations	Meets Expectations	Exceeds Expectations	U/C
1.	Content				
2.	Presentation Skills				
3.	Use of Audio-Visual Aids				
4.	Communication				
5.	Handling Questions				
6.	Audience Management				
7.	References				

Major Positive Feature	
Suggested areas for improvement	Resident's Signature Assessor's Signature

Reflections: Seminar Presentation

Date:...

Article Reference:

What happened?

So what?

What next?

Faculty's Signature

Date...

Seminar Assessment

Date:.................... Topic:.............................

Please rate each criterion. All scores of BE must be justified in the comments box. Write U/C if Unable to Comment/Not Observed.

S. No	Criteria	Below Expectations	Meets Expectations	Exceeds Expectations	U/C
1.	Content				
2.	Presentation Skills				
3.	Use of Audio-Visual Aids				
4.	Communication				
5.	Handling Questions				
6.	Audience Management				
7.	References				

Major Positive Feature	
Suggested areas for improvement	Resident's Signature Assessor's Signature

Reflections: Seminar Presentation

Date:...   Article Reference:
What happened?
So what?
What next?
Faculty's Signature Date..

Seminar Assessment

Date:............................ Topic:.....................................

Please rate each criterion. All scores of BE must be justified in the comments box. Write U/C if Unable to Comment/Not Observed.

S. No	Criteria	Below Expectations	Meets Expectations	Exceeds Expectations	U/C
1.	Content				
2.	Presentation Skills				
3.	Use of Audio-Visual Aids				
4.	Communication				
5.	Handling Questions				
6.	Audience Management				
7.	References				

Major Positive Feature	
Suggested areas for improvement	Resident's Signature Assessor's Signature

Reflections: Seminar Presentation

Date:......................................

Article Reference:

What happened?

So what?

What next?

Faculty's Signature Date..

Seminar Assessment

Date: .... Topic:....................................

Please rate each criterion. All scores of BE must be justified in the comments box. Write U/C if Unable to Comment/Not Observed.

S. No	Criteria	Below Expectations	Meets Expectations	Exceeds Expectations	U/C
1.	Content				
2.	Presentation Skills				
3.	Use of Audio-Visual Aids				
4.	Communication				
5.	Handling Questions				
6.	Audience Management				
7.	References				

Major Positive Feature	
Suggested areas for improvement	Resident's Signature Assessor's Signature

Reflections: Seminar Presentation

Date:....................................

Article Reference:

What happened?

So what?

What next?

Faculty's Signature Date..

(c) Journal Club Assessment

Date:...

Please rate each criterion. All scores of BE must be justified in the comments box. Write U/C if Unable to Comment/Not Observed.

S. No	Criteria	Below Expectations	Meets Expectations	Exceeds Expectations	U/C
1.	Paper Selection (Importance/Relevance)				
2.	Background Knowledge and Introduction of Topic				
3.	Critical Analysis of Methodology				
4.	Critical Analysis of Results				
5.	Conclusions Drawn				
6.	Article Reference (Vancouver Style)				
7.	Audio-Visual Aids				
8.	Handling Questions				
9.	Overall Performance				
Major Positive Feature					

Suggested Areas for Improvement

Criteria	Comments
Article Selection	
Critical Analysis	
Slide Design	
Presentation	
Answering Questions	

Agreed Action Plan	Resident's Signature	Assessor's Signature

(c) Journal Club Assessment

Date:...

Please rate each criterion. All scores of BE must be justified in the comments box. Write U/C if Unable to Comment/Not Observed.

S. No	Criteria	Below Expectations	Meets Expectations	Exceeds Expectations	U/C
1.	Paper Selection (Importance/Relevance)				
2.	Background Knowledge and Introduction of Topic				
3.	Critical Analysis of Methodology				
4.	Critical Analysis of Results				
5.	Conclusions Drawn				
6.	Article Reference (Vancouver Style)				
7.	Audio-Visual Aids				
8.	Handling Questions				
9.	Overall Performance				

Major Positive Feature

Suggested Areas for Improvement

Criteria	Comments
Article Selection	
Critical Analysis	
Slide Design	
Presentation	
Answering Questions	

Agreed Action Plan	Resident's Signature	Assessor's Signature

(c) Journal Club Assessment

Date:...

Please rate each criterion. All scores of BE must be justified in the comments box. Write U/C if Unable to Comment/Not Observed.

S. No	Criteria	Below Expectations	Meets Expectations	Exceeds Expectations	U/C
1.	Paper Selection (Importance/Relevance)				
2.	Background Knowledge and Introduction of Topic				
3.	Critical Analysis of Methodology				
4.	Critical Analysis of Results				
5.	Conclusions Drawn				
6.	Article Reference (Vancouver Style)				
7.	Audio-Visual Aids				
8.	Handling Questions				
9.	Overall Performance				
Major Positive Feature					

Suggested Areas for Improvement

Criteria	Comments
Article Selection	
Critical Analysis	
Slide Design	
Presentation	
Answering Questions	

Agreed Action Plan	Resident's Signature	Assessor's Signature

(c) Journal Club Assessment

Date:...

Please rate each criterion. All scores of BE must be justified in the comments box. Write U/C if Unable to Comment/Not Observed.

S. No	Criteria	Below Expectations	Meets Expectations	Exceeds Expectations	U/C
1.	Paper Selection (Importance/Relevance)				
2.	Background Knowledge and Introduction of Topic				
3.	Critical Analysis of Methodology				
4.	Critical Analysis of Results				
5.	Conclusions Drawn				
6.	Article Reference (Vancouver Style)				
7.	Audio-Visual Aids				
8.	Handling Questions				
9.	Overall Performance				
Major Positive Feature					

Suggested Areas for Improvement

Criteria	Comments
Article Selection	
Critical Analysis	
Slide Design	
Presentation	
Answering Questions	

Agreed Action Plan	Resident's Signature	Assessor's Signature

Reflections

Date:..

Article Reference:

What happened?

So what?

What next?

Faculty's Signature

Date..

Reflections

Date:.. Article Reference:
What happened?
So what?
What next?
Faculty's Signature Date..

Reflections

Date:.......................................
Article Reference:
What happened?
So what?
What next?
Faculty's Signature Date..

Reflections

Date:...
Article Reference:
What happened?
So what?
What next?
Faculty's Signature Date..

III. Workplace Assessment

Mini-CEX Evaluation Summary: First Year

Kindly encircle the relevant dot. Cross the **GRAY** square if not assessed during that encounter.

S. No	Parameter	Setting#										
		Diagnosis										
		Complexity*										
		Grading**	Date	Date	Date	Date	Date	Date	Date	Date	Date	Date
1.	History Taking Skills	E	•	•	•	•	•	•	•	•	•	•
		M	•	•	•	•	•	•	•	•	•	•
		B	•	•	•	•	•	•	•	•	•	•
2.	Physical Examination Skills	E	•	•	•	•	•	•	•	•	•	•
		M	•	•	•	•	•	•	•	•	•	•
		B	•	•	•	•	•	•	•	•	•	•
3.	Humanistic	E	•	•	•	•	•	•	•	•	•	•
	Qualities/Professionalism	M	•	•	•	•	•	•	•	•	•	•
		B	•	•	•	•	•	•	•	•	•	•
4.	Clinical Judgment	E	•	•	•	•	•	•	•	•	•	•
		M	•	•	•	•	•	•	•	•	•	•
		B	•	•	•	•	•	•	•	•	•	•
5.	Counselling Skills/ Communication Skills	E	•	•	•	•	•	•	•	•	•	•
		M	•	•	•	•	•	•	•	•	•	•
		B	•	•	•	•	•	•	•	•	•	•
6.	Organization/Efficiency	E	•	•	•	•	•	•	•	•	•	•
		M	•	•	•	•	•	•	•	•	•	•
		B	•	•	•	•	•	•	•	•	•	•
7.	Overall Clinical Competence	E	•	•	•	•	•	•	•	•	•	•
		M	•	•	•	•	•	•	•	•	•	•
		B	•	•	•	•	•	•	•	•	•	•
Faculty's Signature												

#Setting: O: Outpatient, I: Inpatient, C: Community, E: Emergency

*Complexity: L: Low, M: Moderate, H: High

**Grading: B: Below Expectations, M: Meets Expectations, E: Exceeds Expectations

The mini—CEX form can be downloaded from https://www.abim.org/Media/qlvp1fhb/mini-cex.pdf

Mini-CEX Evaluation Summary: Second Year

Kindly encircle the relevant dot. Cross the **GRAY** square if not assessed during that encounter.

S. No	Parameter	Setting#										
		Diagnosis										
		Complexity*										
		Grading**	Date	Date	Date	Date	Date	Date	Date	Date	Date	Date
1.	History Taking Skills	E	•	•	•	•	•	•	•	•	•	•
		M	•	•	•	•	•	•	•	•	•	•
		B	•	•	•	•	•	•	•	•	•	•
2.	Physical Examination Skills	E	•	•	•	•	•	•	•	•	•	•
		M	•	•	•	•	•	•	•	•	•	•
		B	•	•	•	•	•	•	•	•	•	•
3.	Humanistic	E	•	•	•	•	•	•	•	•	•	•
	Qualities/Professionalism	M	•	•	•	•	•	•	•	•	•	•
		B	•	•	•	•	•	•	•	•	•	•
4.	Clinical Judgment	E	•	•	•	•	•	•	•	•	•	•
		M	•	•	•	•	•	•	•	•	•	•
		B	•	•	•	•	•	•	•	•	•	•
5.	Counselling Skills/ Communication Skills	E	•	•	•	•	•	•	•	•	•	•
		M	•	•	•	•	•	•	•	•	•	•
		B	•	•	•	•	•	•	•	•	•	•
6.	Organization/Efficiency	E	•	•	•	•	•	•	•	•	•	•
		M	•	•	•	•	•	•	•	•	•	•
		B	•	•	•	•	•	•	•	•	•	•
7.	Overall Clinical Competence	E	•	•	•	•	•	•	•	•	•	•
		M	•	•	•	•	•	•	•	•	•	•
		B	•	•	•	•	•	•	•	•	•	•
Faculty's Signature												

#Setting:O: Outpatient, I: Inpatient, C: Community, E: Emergency
*Complexity: L: Low, M: Moderate, H: High
**Grading: B: Below Expectations, M: Meets Expectations, E: Exceeds Expectations

Mini-CEX Evaluation Summary: Third Year

Kindly encircle the relevant dot. Cross the **GRAY** square if not assessed during that encounter.

S. No	Parameter	Setting#										
		Diagnosis										
		Complexity*										
		Grading**	Date	Date	Date	Date	Date	Date	Date	Date	Date	Date
1.	History Taking Skills	E	•	•	•	•	•	•	•	•	•	•
		M	•	•	•	•	•	•	•	•	•	•
		B	•	•	•	•	•	•	•	•	•	•
2.	Physical Examination Skills	E	•	•	•	•	•	•	•	•	•	•
		M	•	•	•	•	•	•	•	•	•	•
		B	•	•	•	•	•	•	•	•	•	•
3.	Humanistic	E	•	•	•	•	•	•	•	•	•	•
	Qualities/Professionalism	M	•	•	•	•	•	•	•	•	•	•
		B	•	•	•	•	•	•	•	•	•	•
4.	Clinical Judgment	E	•	•	•	•	•	•	•	•	•	•
		M	•	•	•	•	•	•	•	•	•	•
		B	•	•	•	•	•	•	•	•	•	•
5.	Counselling Skills/ Communication Skills	E	•	•	•	•	•	•	•	•	•	•
		M	•	•	•	•	•	•	•	•	•	•
		B	•	•	•	•	•	•	•	•	•	•
6.	Organization/Efficiency	E	•	•	•	•	•	•	•	•	•	•
		M	•	•	•	•	•	•	•	•	•	•
		B	•	•	•	•	•	•	•	•	•	•
7.	Overall Clinical Competence	E	•	•	•	•	•	•	•	•	•	•
		M	•	•	•	•	•	•	•	•	•	•
		B	•	•	•	•	•	•	•	•	•	•
Faculty's Signature												

#Setting: O: Outpatient, I: Inpatient, C: Community, E: Emergency
*Complexity: L: Low, M: Moderate, H: High
**Grading: B: Below Expectations, M: Meets Expectations, E: Exceeds Expectations

(B) Directly Observed Procedural Skills (DOPS)

Instructions:
Yearly 6–8 encounters are required for sufficient reliability; however, if required and feasible, more can be undertaken.

Each session should be based on a separate procedure, but can have the same assessor.

The forms used during the sessions should be retained in the departments while the grades be transferred to the summary sheet in the logbook.

DOPS sessions are student driven. The student should proactively try to schedule a session with the concerned teacher.

The DOPS form can be downloaded from https://www.iscp.ac.uk/static/public/DOPSJul2015.pdf

DOPS Assessment Summary: First Year

S. No	Parameter	Procedure										
		Complexity*										
		Grading**	Date	Date	Date	Date	Date	Date	Date	Date	Date	Date
1.	Understanding of Indication(s)/Technique	E	•	•	•	•	•	•	•	•	•	•
		M	•	•	•	•	•	•	•	•	•	•
		B	•	•	•	•	•	•	•	•	•	•
2.	Informed Consent Obtained	E	•	•	•	•	•	•	•	•	•	•
		M	•	•	•	•	•	•	•	•	•	•
		B	•	•	•	•	•	•	•	•	•	•
3.	Appropriate Pre-procedure Preparation	E	•	•	•	•	•	•	•	•	•	•
		M	•	•	•	•	•	•	•	•	•	•
		B	•	•	•	•	•	•	•	•	•	•
4.	Appropriate Analgesia/ Safe Sedation	E	•	•	•	•	•	•	•	•	•	•
		M	•	•	•	•	•	•	•	•	•	•
		B	•	•	•	•	•	•	•	•	•	•
5.	Technical Ability	E	•	•	•	•	•	•	•	•	•	•
		M	•	•	•	•	•	•	•	•	•	•
		B	•	•	•	•	•	•	•	•	•	•
6.	Aseptic Technique	E	•	•	•	•	•	•	•	•	•	•
		M	•	•	•	•	•	•	•	•	•	•
		B	•	•	•	•	•	•	•	•	•	•
7.	Seeks Help where Appropriate	E	•	•	•	•	•	•	•	•	•	•
		M		•								•
		B	•	•	•	•	•	•	•	•	•	•
8.	Post-Procedure Management	E	•	•	•	•	•	•	•	•	•	•
		M	•	•	•	•	•	•	•	•	•	•
		B	•	•	•	•	•	•	•	•	•	•
9.	Communication Skills	E	•	•	•	•	•	•	•	•	•	•
		M	•	•	•	•	•	•	•	•	•	•
		B	•	•	•	•	•	•	•	•	•	•
10.	Professionalism/ Consideration of Patient	E	•	•	•	•	•	•	•	•	•	•
		M	•	•	•	•	•	•	•	•	•	•
		B	•	•	•	•	•	•	•	•	•	•
11.	Overall Ability to Perform	E	•	•	•	•	•	•	•	•	•	•
	Procedure	M	•	•	•	•	•	•	•	•	•	•
		B	•	•	•	•	•	•	•	•	•	•
Faculty's Signature												

Kindly encircle the relevant dot. Cross the gray square if not assessed during that encounter

* Complexity:
L: Low
M: Moderate
H: High

** Grading:
B: Below Expectations
M: Meets Expectations
E: Exceeds Expectations

DOPS Assessment Summary: Second Year

S. No	Parameter	Procedure										
		Complexity*										
		Grading**	Date	Date	Date	Date	Date	Date	Date	Date	Date	Date
1.	Understanding of Indication(s)/Technique	E	•	•	•	•	•	•	•	•	•	•
		M	•	•	•	•	•	•	•	•	•	•
		B	•	•	•	•	•	•	•	•	•	•
2.	Informed Consent Obtained	E	•	•	•	•	•	•	•	•	•	•
		M	•	•	•	•	•	•	•	•	•	•
		B	•	•	•	•	•	•	•	•	•	•
3.	Appropriate Pre-procedure Preparation	E	•	•	•	•	•	•	•	•	•	•
		M	•	•	•	•	•	•	•	•	•	•
		B	•	•	•	•	•	•	•	•	•	•
4.	Appropriate Analgesia/ Safe Sedation	E	•	•	•	•	•	•	•	•	•	•
		M	•	•	•	•	•	•	•	•	•	•
		B	•	•	•	•	•	•	•	•	•	•
5.	Technical Ability	E	•	•	•	•	•	•	•	•	•	•
		M	•	•	•	•	•	•	•	•	•	•
		B	•	•	•	•	•	•	•	•	•	•
6.	Aseptic Technique	E	•	•	•	•	•	•	•	•	•	•
		M	•	•	•	•	•	•	•	•	•	•
		B	•	•	•	•	•	•	•	•	•	•
7.	Seeks Help where Appropriate	E	•	•	•	•	•	•	•	•	•	•
		M		•								•
		B	•	•	•	•	•	•	•	•	•	•
8.	Post-Procedure Management	E	•	•	•	•	•	•	•	•	•	•
		M	•	•	•	•	•	•	•	•	•	•
		B	•	•	•	•	•	•	•	•	•	•
9.	Communication Skills	E	•	•	•	•	•	•	•	•	•	•
		M	•	•	•	•	•	•	•	•	•	•
		B	•	•	•	•	•	•	•	•	•	•
10.	Professionalism/ Consideration of Patient	E	•	•	•	•	•	•	•	•	•	•
		M	•	•	•	•	•	•	•	•	•	•
		B	•	•	•	•	•	•	•	•	•	•
11.	Overall Ability to Perform	E	•	•	•	•	•	•	•	•	•	•
	Procedure	M	•	•	•	•	•	•	•	•	•	•
		B	•	•	•	•	•	•	•	•	•	•
Faculty's Signature												

Kindly encircle the relevant dot. Cross the gray square if not assessed during that encounter

*Complexity:
L: Low
M: Moderate
H: High

** Grading:
B: Below Expectations
M: Meets Expectations
E: Exceeds Expectations

DOPS Assessment Summary: Third Year

S. No	Parameter											
		Procedure										
		Complexity*										
S. No	Parameter	Grading**	Date	Date	Date	Date	Date	Date	Date	Date	Date	Date
1.	Understanding of Indication(s)/Technique	E										
		M										
		B										
2.	Informed Consent Obtained	E										
		M										
		B										
3.	Appropriate Pre-procedure Preparation	E										
		M										
		B										
4.	Appropriate Analgesia/ Safe Sedation	E										
		M										
		B										
5.	Technical Ability	E										
		M										
		B										
6.	Aseptic Technique	E										
		M										
		B										
7.	Seeks Help where Appropriate	E										
		M										
		B										
8.	Post-Procedure Management	E										
		M										
		B										
9.	Communication Skills	E										
		M										
		B										
10.	Professionalism/ Consideration of Patient	E										
		M										
		B										
11.	Overall Ability to Perform	E										
	Procedure	M										
		B										
Faculty's Signature												

Kindly encircle the relevant dot. Cross the gray square if not assessed during that encounter

*Complexity:
L: Low
M: Moderate
H: High

** Grading:
B: Below Expectations
M: Meets Expectations
E: Exceeds Expectations

Summary of Procedures

S. No	Date	Procedure	Observed/Assisted/Performed	Trainer's Signature

IV. Research Skills

Thesis

Thesis Title:..

Supervisor:..

Co-Supervisor(s):...

Activity	Date of Completion	Remarks	Thesis Supervisor's Signature
Thesis Protocol			
Departmental Protocol Presentation Research Committee Approval Ethics Committee Approval/Number			
Review of Literature			
Data Collection			
Statistical Analysis			
Interim Results Presentation			
Completion			
Others			

Activity	Details	Date	Faculty's Signature
Training Received in Research Methods Thesis and/or Protocol Writing Paper Writing Medical Education Technology Literature Search			
Poster Presentation			
Research Paper Presentation			
Publication(s)			
Research Projects			
Others			

VI. Teaching

Activity	Date	Topic	Rating (B/M/E)	Faculty's Signature
Undergraduates				
Paramedical Staff				
Parents/Patients' Attendants				

VI. Self-directed Learning

Topic:

Objectives:

Task:

Methodology:

VI. Self-directed Learning

Topic:

Objectives:

Task:

Methodology:

VI. Self-directed Learning

Topic:

Objectives:

Task:

Methodology:

VI. Self-directed Learning

Topic:

Objectives:

Task:

Methodology:

Reflections: Self-directed Learning

<table>
<tr><td>S. No</td><td>Topic:.. Date:......................................

Specific Objective:</td></tr>
<tr><td colspan="2">What happened?</td></tr>
<tr><td colspan="2">So what?</td></tr>
<tr><td colspan="2">What next?</td></tr>
<tr><td colspan="2">Faculty's Signature Date:...</td></tr>
</table>

Reflections: Self-directed Learning

<table>
<tr><td>S. No</td><td>Topic:.. Date:......................................

Specific Objective:</td></tr>
<tr><td colspan="2">What happened?</td></tr>
<tr><td colspan="2">So what?</td></tr>
<tr><td colspan="2">What next?</td></tr>
<tr><td colspan="2">Faculty's Signature Date:...</td></tr>
</table>

Reflections: Self-directed Learning

<table>
<tr><td>S. No</td><td>Topic:.. Date:....................................

Specific Objective:</td></tr>
<tr><td colspan="2">What happened?</td></tr>
<tr><td colspan="2">So what?</td></tr>
<tr><td colspan="2">What next?</td></tr>
<tr><td colspan="2">Faculty's Signature Date:..</td></tr>
</table>

Reflections: Self-directed Learning

<table>
<tr><td>S. No</td><td>Topic:.. Date:.......................................

Specific Objective:</td></tr>
<tr><td colspan="2">What happened?</td></tr>
<tr><td colspan="2">So what?</td></tr>
<tr><td colspan="2">What next?</td></tr>
<tr><td colspan="2">Faculty's Signature Date:...</td></tr>
</table>

Participation in Departmental Activities

Activity	Details of Event	Date	Faculty's Signature
Participation in Community Health Activities			
Participation in Conferences/ Workshops and Role			
Participation in IAP/Other Quiz			
Others			

Professionalism, Ethics and Communication Skills

Professionalism Skills: First Year

<table>
<tr><td>S. No</td><td>Setting: Inpatient/Outpatient: Date:..................................</td></tr>
<tr><td colspan="2">Difficult Doctor-Patient Encounter: What happened?</td></tr>
<tr><td colspan="2">How was it handled?</td></tr>
<tr><td colspan="2">Outcome</td></tr>
<tr><td colspan="2">Faculty's Signature Date:...</td></tr>
</table>

Professionalism Skills: Second Year

S. No	Setting: Inpatient/Outpatient: Date:....................................
Difficult Doctor-Patient Encounter: What happened?	
How was it handled?	
Outcome	
Faculty's Signature Date:..	

Professionalism Skills: Third Year

S. No	Setting: Inpatient/Outpatient: Date:..................................
Difficult Doctor-Patient Encounter: What happened?	
How was it handled?	
Outcome	
Faculty's Signature	Date:..

Professionalism Mini Evaluation Exercise (P-MEX) Assessment Summary

S. No	Parameter	Encounter	1	2	3	4	5	6	7	8	9
		Scenario* (R/S)									
		Residency Year									
		Grading**	Date	Date	Date	Date	Date	Date	Date	Date	Date
1.	Doctor-Patient Relationshi p Skills	E									
		M									
		B									
2.	Reflective Skills	E									
		M									
		B									
3.	Time Management	E									
		M									
		B									
4.	Inter-Professional Relationship Skills	E									
		M									
		B									
Faculty's Signature											

Miscellaneous

Activity	Details	Date	Faculty's Signature
Participation in Webinars/Conferences/ CMEs and Role			
Awards Received			
Administrative Work			
Others			

TESTIMONIALS

TESTIMONIALS

TESTIMONIALS

Term	Description
Agreed Action Plan	Mutually agreed (between trainer and trainee) method for identifying needs, establishing goals and developing strategies to reach those goals.
Assessment	Assessment is the process of gathering and discussing information from multiple and diverse sources in order to develop a deep understanding of what the trainee know, understand, and can do with their knowledge as a result of their educational experiences; the process culminates when assessment results are used to improve subsequent learning.
Direct Observation of Procedural Skills (DOPS)	DOPS is a structured assessment for students on their practical procedure competency as well as communication skills with the patient. The time allocated depends on the length of the procedure to be carried out followed by 5 minutes of verbal feedback by the assessor. The checklist has an emphasis on patient safety and professionalism. The observation is recorded on a standard form and immediate feedback is provided to the resident. Each competency on the form is assessed individually and no mean is taken.
mini-Clinical Evaluation Exercise (m-CEX)	A mini-CEX encounter consists of a single faculty member observing a resident while that resident conducts a focused history and physical examination. It is a workplace based formative assessment of core clinical skills by direct observation or "snapshot" of a trainee-patient interaction and is intended to be a short (about 20 minutes) encounter. The observation is recorded on a standard form and immediate feedback is provided to the resident. Each competency on the form is assessed individually and no mean is taken.

NOTES

NOTES

NOTES